Thyroid Disease

The Ultimate Handbook for Naturally Managing your Hyperthyroidism or Hypothyroidism (and be normal)

Table of Contents

Introduction

Chapter 1: Thyroid Gland and Thyroid Gland Functions

Chapter 2: Main Symptoms of Thyroid Disease

Chapter 3: Types of Thyroid Diseases and Disorders

Chapter 4: Causes of Major Thyroid Diseases

Chapter 5: Ways to Naturally Treat Hypothyroidism and Hyperthyroidism

Chapter 6: Natural Ways to Prevent Thyroid Diseases

Conclusion

Introduction

I want to thank you as well as congratulate you for downloading the book, *"Thyroid Disease"*. I've lived the majority of my life with this disease and I'm happy to say that after many years of struggling, I'm now living an Amazing life. I really wanted to share the successful strategies and techniques that I used to obtain freedom from my condition so I can help other people.

This book contains proven steps and strategies on how to become truly healthy through easy natural remedies and simple lifestyle despite having a thyroid condition or disease.

Here's an inescapable fact: you need to learn to take control of your thyroid condition now. This means more than taking medications on a daily basis. This means managing different aspects of your diet and lifestyle to ensure that you continue to live a fulfilled and rewarding life.

Not taking control of your condition will mean that you will inevitably be at it's mercy. Thyroid disease should not become you. You need to ensure that you rise to the challenge, put in place measures to life processes to stamp out it's hindrance on your life and start living the life you always wanted. Now.

It's time for you to become a healthy person by just following the basic steps and knowledge that lies within these pages. A healthy you is just around the corner with the aid of these exciting, practical and healthy practices.

I really hope to meet the new you sometime in the near future.

Chapter 1: Thyroid Gland and Thyroid Gland Functions

In order to understand Thyroid disease we must first understand how it works and how it effects your body. Lets take a look at some of the core concepts first and then we will move on to how to easily control them.

Thyroid Gland

The thyroid gland is an important gland in our body. It is butterfly-shaped and sits low in the front of your neck. The thyroid gland lies underneath the Adam's apple and along the front side of your windpipe. The thyroid gland includes two side lobes and they are connected by the isthmus, which is a bridge located in the middle.

When your thyroid gland is in normal size, you are unable to feel it with your hands. It is brownish with a red tint due to being full of blood vessels. There are also nerves, which are extremely important for the quality of voice as it passes through the thyroid gland.

Thyroid Gland Functions

The thyroid gland secretes many different hormones. As a collective group, these hormones are called the thyroid hormones. The hormone **thyroxine** is the main hormone and is also referred to as **T4**.

The hormones secreted by the thyroid gland act through the entire body. They influence a person's growth and development, metabolism, and even body temperature.

Appropriate amounts of the thyroid hormones are crucial for brain development in infancy as well as in childhood.

Chapter 2: Main Symptoms of Thyroid Disease

Main Symptoms of Thyroid Diseases

Weight Loss or Gain: If you loose or gain weight unexpectedly with no explanation, then it can be a sign of thyroid gland problems. If you gain weight, this could be a sign of low levels of the hormone produced by the thyroid gland. On the other hand, if you experience rapid weight loss you are experiencing high levels of the hormone. This is a sign of hyperthyroidism. This will affect those with the condition regardless if they are trying to lose or gain weight.

Neck Swelling: If you find that your neck is swollen or is enlarged, this is a visual clue that there may be an issue with your thyroid gland. It could be a goiter that can cause either hyperthyroidism or hypothyroidism. In some cases, this maybe a sign of nodules or cancer.

Heart Rate Changes: The hormones produced by the thyroid gland affects the body and can influence how the heart beats. Those with hypothyroidism might notice a drop in their heart rate. Hyperthyroidism, on the other hand, will cause the heart rate to increase. It may also increase blood pressure, as well as cause the sensation of a pounding heart or heart palpitations.

Changes in Mood or Energy: There is a disorder that causes a very noticeable mood or energy level change. Hypothyroidism causes people to feel sluggish, tired, and often times depressed. Hyperthyroidism will cause sleeping problems, restlessness, irritability, and in some cases it will also cause anxiety. This will affect your daily life with work, family, and even leisure time.

Loss of Hair: Often times the person afflicted with hypothyroidism or hyperthyroidism will experience extreme hair loss. Most of those who experience this will grow their hair back once the condition has been addressed. This can be a depressing situation though, especially if the one suffering is a female.

Feelings of Being Too Hot or Too Cold: Having a thyroid disorder can often times disrupt the body's capability to regulate its temperature. Those with hypothyroidism may feel unusually cold while those who are experiencing hyperthyroidism will find that they are often times hot. They may even sweat a lot and have an aversion to heat. This is refered to as *extreme change*. For instance, there maybe people who are just sitting around you and they seem to be just fine with the temperature of the room. You, on the other hand, seem to need a coat suited for the Antarctic or a personal heater to heat things up.

Hypothyroidism Symptoms

Hypothyroidism is a condition wherein the **thyroid gland does not produce enough thyroid hormone (T4)**. There are other symptoms for hypothyroidism, which are not included above. Along with the main symptoms of this thyroid condition, there are other smaller and less obvious symptoms that a person with hypothyroidism may experience. These would include brittle nails, dry skin, numbness of the hands, tingling in the hands, constipation, and unusual menstrual periods

Hyperthyroidism Symptoms

Hyperthyroidism is a condition wherein the **thyroid gland over produces the thyroid hormone (T4)**. Some of the minor symptoms that people with hyperthyroidism display include weakness in the muscles, trembling hands, problems with vision, diarrhea, and unusual menstrual periods (cycle may be irregular.)

Thyroid Disease Tests

If you feel that you may have an issue with your thyroid gland, it is would be essential that tests be performed to ensure that it is actually your thyroid gland and not any another underlying condition. Here are typical tests that may be performed should your thyroid be a suspect of your health condition.

Anti-TPO Antibodies: When you are subject to an autoimmune disease, proteins attack the thyroid peroxidase enzyme mistakenly. This can cause other conditions in the long run if this goes untreated. This test shows the anti-bodies that are present in your blood.

Thyroid Scan: This test is where a tiny amount of radioactive iodine is given orally in order to get pictures of the thyroid gland. The radioactive iodine works its way to the thyroid gland, allowing it to be visible when observed through the scanner.

Thyroid Biopsy: The thyroid biopsy test is performed by having a small amount of the thyroid gland tissue removed. It is done in order to look for the thyroid gland cancer. This is typically performed using a biopsy needle.

Thyroid Stimulating Hormone – TSH: This hormone is secreted by your brain. TSH is in charge of regulating thyroid hormone release. This is typically given in pill form. The medication will include this hormone to help the production of the other hormones.

Thyroxine T3 and T4: This is checked by having a blood test done. These primarily make up the thyroid hormone. The main hormone of the thyroid is T4.

Thyroglobulins: This is secreted by the thyroid gland and is used as a marker for thyroid cancer. High levels of this hormone may indicate a possibility of thyroid cancer.

Other Tests: There are some other tests that can help identify the growth of thyroid cancer. These tests include MRI scans, PET scans, or CT scans.

Typical Treatments for Thyroid Diseases

These diseases and conditions can be scary situations. There are treatments available to help ease or eradicate such condition or disease. Here is a list of the typical treatments that are offered for thyroid gland problems.

Thyroidectomy (Surgery): This treatment is performed by a surgeon. They will remove all the parts of the thyroid during the operation. Thyroidectomy is performed when the patient has a goiter, cancer, or hyperthyroidism.

Antithyroid Medications: These medications slow down the production of the thyroid hormone that causes hyperthyroidism. There are two common medications under this category. These medications are called propylthiouracil and methimazole.

External Radiation: This is a beam of radiation, which is directed towards the thyroid. It is carried out over a series of appointments. The high-energy ray will kill the cancer cells located in the thyroid gland.

Radioactive Iodine: This is iodine that includes radioactivity and is used in small doses in order to test the gland or eradicate an overactive thyroid gland. There are large doses given to those who are experiencing thyroid cancer.

Thyroid Hormone Medication: This is a treatment followed out daily and replaces the hormone when the patient is no longer able to produce the hormone on his or her own. This pill is used to treat hypothyroidism and will help prevent some thyroid cancers.

Hypothyroidism Treatment

This is one of the main issues an individual has with their thyroid gland. Hypothyroidism is when the thyroid gland does not produce enough of the thyroid hormones for the body to function on a normal basis. Once diagnosed the patient will more than likely be put on a daily medication in the form of a pill. The pill will lead to a noticeable improvement after just a couple of weeks of taking the medication daily.

Long-term treatments will result in an increase in energy, lowered levels of cholesterol, and weight loss. Most of those who suffer from hypothyroidism need to take medication to replace the thyroid hormones for the rest of their lives.

Hyperthyroidism Treatment

This is the other known issue that individuals suffer from. With hyperthyroidism, their thyroid gland becomes over active. The thyroid gland over produces the thyroid hormone and affects that body in ways that makes daily life difficult. This condition is treated with medication that lowers the amount of hormones that is produced by the thyroid gland.

This specific condition may go away eventually. However, there are many individuals that will remain on the specified medication on a long-term basis. Some medications are prescribed to alleviate the symptoms of hyperthyroidism. These other medications address symptoms like tremors and rapid pulse.

Another option that patients can opt for include radioactive iodine. This destroys the thyroid gland over a certain amount of time. The time span is about 6 to 18 weeks. Once the thyroid gland is destroyed or removed using surgical measures, most individuals will have to take thyroid hormones in the form of medication.

Thyroid Disorder Surgery

If an individual is suffering from hyperthyroidism and the medication that is prescribed does not work, then the individual will more than likely undergo surgery. This surgery is also done for goiters and nodules. Should the surgery be completed for the purpose of removing the gland, then the patient will have to take thyroid hormones to normalize their bodily functions that the gland is responsible for daily.

Chapter 3: Types of Thyroid Diseases and Conditions

As you can see, the thyroid gland is an important part of functioning normally. It has influence over your entire body. A few of the bodily functions that the thyroid is responsible for are the loss or gain of weight, metabolism, energy levels, and more. It can cause different reactions depending on the disease, condition, or disorder. Some sufferers find it hard to lead a normal daily life due to certain health situations dealing with the thyroid gland. You can learn about the diseases, conditions, and disorders here.

When a thyroid disorder is left untreated, the possibility of having increased cholesterol levels would be high. This will in turn raise your risk of having stroke or heart attack. In some more severe cases, having low thyroid gland hormones can cause a life threatening decrease to your body temperature and loss of consciousness. When a victim of hyperthyroidism goes untreated, they will also have serious heart issues and their bones will become brittle.

Thyroid Diseases

Hyperthyroidism: This happens when there is an excessive amount of thyroid hormones being produced. It is typically caused by the disease called Graves or caused by an overactive nodule in the thyroid gland.

Hypothyroidism: This is when too little of the thyroid hormone is produced. This can be a caused by the thyroid gland being damaged from an autoimmune disease.

Graves: This is a disease, which is considered to be an autoimmune condition. This condition may bring about hyperthyroidism. This disease forces the body to produce antibodies that attack the thyroid gland, as well as the viruses and bacteria just as they are supposed to. At times, the thyroid gland will even be removed due to this disease.

Thyroid Cancer: This is not a common form of cancer. It typically is curable with different treatments like surgery, hormone treatments, or radiation. The thyroid gland is usually removed due to the cancer and the patient is then put on hypothyroidism medication to replace the hormone levels they are no longer able to produce.

Thyroid Conditions

Goiter: This is a term generalized for the swelling of the thyroid gland. They are at times harmless; however, other times can represent another condition. One condition that this could be a result from is iodine deficiency. Another is Hashimoto's thyroiditis, which is also an inflammation of the thyroid gland.

Thyroiditis: Thyroiditis is considered to be an inflammation of the gland. It is typically caused by an autoimmune condition or a viral infection. This condition can be quite painful, but at times can cause no symptoms at all.

Thyroid Nodule: This is considered to be a lump or mass found in the thyroid. This is a common occurrence and few of the nodules are cancerous. At times, the thyroid nodule will secrete an excess amount of the thyroid hormones. This causes hyperthyroidism.

Thyroid Storm: This is not a well-known condition. This is a rare type of hyperthyroidism. It is caused by an extremely high level of thyroid hormones and will cause severe sickness.

Mistaken Menopause

Women are more common to have an issue with their thyroid gland than men. If the affected person is that of a mature age, symptoms can be mistaken for the pre-stages of menopause. Due to the thyroid disorder symptoms like changes in the menstrual period, some women have mistakenly thought the thyroid disorder was the onset of menopause. Should the woman suspect the issues to be due to her thyroid gland, a simple blood test can be done to affirm or discredit it.

Chapter 4: Causes of Major Thyroid Diseases

Just as other diseases or disorders, there are multiple causes. Here is a list of causes of thyroid gland conditions. This list may help pinpoint issues that you typically would not be aware of under normal circumstances.

Graves' Disease

This is caused by the **malfunction in your body's immune system**. The exact cause of this condition is still unknown. One of the main responses of the immune system is to produce antibodies. These antibodies are made to target bacteria, viruses, or other foreign substances.

The thyroid function is maintained by a hormone that is secreted by a small gland at the base of your brain called the **pituitary gland**. The antibody, which is associated with Graves' disease, called TRAb (thyrotropin receptor antibody), acts as the regulatory pituitary hormone. This means that the TRAb hormone overrides the typical regulation put forth by the thyroid. This causes an overproduction of the hormones made by the thyroid gland - hence, hyperthyroidism occurs.

This certain condition is known to be caused by a buildup of carbohydrates in the patient's skin. The cause of buildup is unknown. It seems as though the same antibody causes thyroid dysfunction and also effects the surrounding of the eyes.

Graves' disease typically appears simultaneously or several months after a patient is diagnosed with hyperthyroidism. There are symptoms and signs that may show years before, and at times after, the onset of the thyroid condition hyperthyroidism.

Toxic Adenoma

Toxic adenoma is a disorder that happens when a **growth of a nodule occurs**. The nodules secrete hormones, which causes problems in your body. Typically the nodules are not cancerous, although they may spread through the body or multiply. It is extended past the pituitary gland and combines with follicular cells in order to form and make hormones on a larger scale. Once the secretion reaches over the normal amount of hormones, the patient suffers from hyperthyroidism. Toxic adenomas constitute almost 2% of the hyperthyroidism cases.

Toxic adenomas are found more in women than in men. There are cases when patients will need to get the nodule analyzed and tested immediately. The nodule will be identified through physical examination, as well as radiographic images. These tests will help in pinpointing the toxic adenoma. In some situations, the tests will also reveal thyrotoxicosis. These specific nodules are dark in color and scanning will help view them better.

Typically, toxic adenoma is treated easily by medications; however, surgery is also a treatment that is sought after once the condition seems unresponsive to medications. Most of the anti-thyroid medications will help in lowering the hormones produced by the thyroid gland. Once the sufferer is taken off of the medication, they are considered to be in the stages of recovery.

Thyroid Nodules

Thyroid nodules are classified as small growths or lumps that occur inside the thyroid gland. They are typically located in the front part of the neck located below the Adam's apple. There are many causes for nodules. These growths or nodules are typically benign and non-cancerous. However, they do tend to spread and multiply. This condition is found more so in women than in men.

As a person **matures in age**, the chances of forming thyroid nodules increase. Over time the nodules may become cancerous. This is typically the case when the nodule is hard or if the nodule is attached to the organs that surround it.

It is also proven that if the **family has a history of nodules**, it is passed down to other generations. The condition called *medullary thyroid carcinoma* can be passed down as well and cause thyroid problems. In this case the affected individual will experience difficulty breathing. Should the person be younger than 20 years of age or older than 70 years of age, then the person will experience nodules.

Thyroid nodules can also occur due to a **deficiency of iodine or Hashimoto's disease**. Those who experience this condition will find that they have pressure around and in their necks. Other symptoms that occurs along with the nodules is hoarseness, pain in the neck, difficulty while swallowing, nervousness, increased appetite, weight loss, restlessness, skin blushing, skin flushing, and more. Those who have nodules and have hypothyroidism will face other symptoms as well.

Subacute Thyroiditis

Subacute thyroiditis refers to an inflamed thyroid. In most cases, thyroiditis does not cause pain located in the gland;

however, it does normally lead to either hypothyroidism or hyperthyroidism. Both of these conditions cause symptoms along the lines of weight changes, fatigue, and anxiety.

This specific thyroid problem causes discomfort and pain inside the thyroid gland. Those with this specific condition will also experience symptoms of an overactive thyroid and later will experience symptoms of an underactive gland.

Subacute thyroiditis typically **happens after the patient experiences an upper respiratory viral infection like mumps or flu**. When an individual has mumps, it is highly contagious and causes swollen salivary glands. Although subacute thyroiditis is rare, it is more common in middle aged women.

This condition is found by performing blood tests. The tests will not only show if an individual has subacute thyroiditis, but it will also tell what stage the patient is in with their condition.

Hypothyroidism

Hypothyroidism is a condition in which your thyroid gland does not produce enough thyroid hormones for your body to function normally. Without the balance of hormones, your body will not be able to function to the fullest. There are quite a few causes of hypothyroidism.

One cause of hypothyroidism can be attributed to an **autoimmune disease**. Those who developed a specific inflammatory disorder called **Hashimoto's thyroiditis** will also experience hypothyroidism. The autoimmune disorders happen when the patient's immune system creates antibodies that wage war on their own bodily tissues. In many cases, the war is on the thyroid gland as well. It is not known exactly why the body produces antibodies that attack the gland. Some scientists believed it is a genetic flaw. Autoimmune diseases do result in more than one factor.

Hyperthyroidism treatment can also be attributed to hypothyroidism. Those who produce an overload of thyroid hormones are treated with a medication known as *radioactive iodine* or by *anti-thyroid medication* in order to reduce the amount of hormone levels they produce. In some cases, treatment for hyperthyroidism can result in a permanent condition of hypothyroidism.

Thyroid surgery is another cause of hypothyroidism. When a surgeon removes a part of the thyroid gland, it can diminish or even stop the production of thyroid hormones. This is a direct cause of hypothyroidism.

Radiation therapy is another cause of the condition hypothyroidism. The radiation that is used to treat different types of cancer of the neck or head can affect the thyroid gland. It can lead to hypothyroidism.

Certain medications can also cause hypothyroidism. Many medications that include lithium can cause this condition. Medications that are used to treat psychiatric disorders have been known to contribute to the count of hypothyroidism inflicted individuals.

Congenital disease is a condition that some infants are born with. It is a defective thyroid gland or even no thyroid gland present in the neck. In this case the thyroid gland was not developed normally or at all and this condition has no known causes. This will cause hypothyroidism in the child. Screenings are done to ensure the child grows normally.

Pituitary disorder is a rare cause, but does cause hypothyroidism. It is the failure of the pituitary gland. The gland does no produce enough hormones that stimulate the thyroid gland. This thyroid-stimulating hormone is called TSH (thyroid stimulating hormone). It is typically caused by a benign tumor located in the pituitary gland.

Pregnancy is also one of the known causes for hypothyroidism. Some pregnant women develop this condition during or even after pregnancy; postpartum hypothyroidism. It is due to the production of antibodies that attack the thyroid. If this is left untreated, the woman will endure an increased risk of miscarriage, pre-eclampsia, or premature delivery. It also is responsible for increasing the woman's blood pressure during the last trimester of the pregnancy. In some cases this can affect the fetus.

Iodine deficiency can cause hypothyroidism. Iodine is a trace mineral found in seaweed, seafood, and plants that are grown in iodine enriched soils. It is extremely important for the production of the thyroid hormone. In certain parts of the world, this condition is well known. This problem has been addressed in the United States with iodine infused salt. Should an individual take in too much iodine, they will also cause hypothyroidism.

It is noted that those who experience hypothyroidism may experience more serious consequences if left untreated. Going long-term without treatment can result in **myxedema coma**. It is a rare condition, yet it is also fatal and will require an immediate hormone treatment.

Hyperthyroidism

There are numerous causes of hyperthyroidism. Some of the other conditions actually end in hyperthyroidism like Graves' disease, Plummer's disease, toxic adenoma, and thyroiditis.

Graves' disease is an autoimmune disorder in which the sufferer will produce antibodies that attack the thyroid. This is the most common cause for hyperthyroidism. Typically the antibodies are to fight off foreign substances, bacteria, and viruses. Unfortunately, Graves' disease puts out the antibodies that attack the thyroid and hyperthyroidism is one of the side effects of this condition. The thyroid is removed and then the individual will experience hypothyroidism.

Toxic adenoma, Plummer's disease, and multi-nodular goiters also cause hyperthyroidism. This happens when one or more of the adenomas located in your thyroid produce too much of the thyroid hormone called T4. An adenoma is part of the thyroid gland that walls itself away from the rest of the thyroid gland. It forms a non-cancerous, benign lump that will enlarge the thyroid gland. Not all of the adenomas produce an excess amount of T4; however, doctors are still unsure as to why this is a factor in producing too much T4.

Thyroiditis happens when your thyroid gland is inflamed for reasons unknown. The inflammation will cause an excess of hormones to be stored inside the gland and will leak into the bloodstream. One type of thyroiditis that is rare is known as subacute thyroiditis. It tends to cause pain in the gland. Other types of thyroiditis are painless and can occur after a woman gives birth.

Hashimoto's Thyroiditis

Hashimoto's disease is considered to be an autoimmune disorder. This is where your immune system produces antibodies that end up damaging your thyroid. It is unsure of why the body produces these antibodies that attack the gland. There are some scientists that believe a virus or even a bacteria may trigger this response. Other scientists believe that a genetic flaw causes it. However, there is a combination of different factors such as heredity, age, and gender that may be a determination of whether or not an individual will develop this disease.

Thyroid Gland Removal

The thyroid gland may at times cause a condition known as hyperthyroidism. Hyperthyroidism is the overproduction of the thyroid hormones. When medication does not work, some individuals will undergo surgery in order to remove the thyroid. This in turn will cause hypothyroidism and the individual will be placed on daily medication in order to balance out the hormone levels in their body.

Excessive Amounts of Iodide

There are over-the-counter medicines that include to much iodide. These medicines are made for colds and sinus problems. Other situations that will offer too much iodide is amiodarone, which is a heart medication, or certain dyes given for x-rays. Those who have too much iodide may experience hypothyroidism.

Lithium

This specific drug is related to cases of hypothyroidism.

Chapter 5: Ways to Naturally Treat Hypothyroidism and Hyperthyroidism

Hypothyroidism

The thyroid gland is an important part of your body. It is located in your neck and is the shape of a butterfly located below the Adam's apple. It controls your metabolism, other hormones, weight changes, body temperature, and more. It is a fundamental and complex gland that helps keep your entire body balanced.

Hypothyroidism, also known as low *thyroid function*. This happens when an individual experiences low hormone levels produced by their thyroid gland. According to different medical doctors hypothyroidism is a silent epidemic. It is affecting more people than originally thought. The symptoms can go unnoticed for years until a major symptom rears its head. Often times the hypothyroidism is due to another health condition rather than the thyroid gland.

According to Doctor Datis Kharrazian, 90% of individuals that experience hypothyroidism actually have Hashimoto's disease. This is a disease in which antibodies are made to attack the thyroid gland and not just viruses and bacteria.

Fortunately, there are ways to help you without getting pricked, prodded, and x-rayed. Natural ways exist for putting your own body back into balance. Of course just like any new regimen, it does take time to get used to the changes. Just remember that it take threes weeks to break a habit, and three weeks to make a new one. Follow these guidelines to help aid your body in repairs.

Sugar and Caffeine: Yes, you were probably scared this was going to be mentioned. Life is busy and at times we all fall into the *"need energy aid"* traps. These are unnatural chemicals that you are introducing into your body and although it does help for the moment, you are hurting your body in the long haul. You will need to reduce or even eliminate caffeine and sugar in your diet. This includes refined carbohydrates. An example of refined carbohydrates is flour. Flour is treated like sugar by your body. You can eat as many non-starchy vegetables as you would like, but limit refined carbs, sugar, and caffeine.

More Protein: Protein is extremely important. It helps transport T4 (thyroid hormone) to all of the body's tissues. Eating protein helps normalize the functions of the thyroid gland. Proteins that you should include in your diet are nuts, nut butters, meats, eggs, fish, quinoa, and legumes.

More Fat: Alright, this may sound like it goes against every healthy diet tip given. However, the term moderation plays the key roll in this requirement. Eating low levels of fat and cholesterol can cause a hormonal imbalance. Natural fats that are a great source of these needs are flax seeds, fish, nuts, nut butters, olive oil, ghee, avocados, cheese, yogurt, cottage cheese, and coconut milk items.

More Nutrients: It is a great idea to take a daily vitamin. Vitamin levels are important when wanting to normalize your hormone levels. Nutrients that will help keep your body balanced include iron, vitamin D, omega-3 fatty acids, zinc, copper, selenium, all B vitamins, vitamin A, and iodine.

Go Gluten Free: Those with Hashimoto's disease should stay away from gluten. Gluten has the same properties as the thyroid gland and will cause the condition to attack the gland more aggressively.

Goitrogens: Stay away from too many goitrogens. They will interfere with the functions of the thyroid gland. Although the foods are very healthy for you, it is best to eat them in moderation. Goitrogens foods include Brussels sprouts, broccoli, cabbage, kale, cauliflower, kohlrabi, turnips, rutabaga, millet, strawberries, spinach, peaches, peanuts, watercress, radishes, and soybeans. Fortunately, cooking these foods will inactivate the goitrogenic compounds. It is more so caused by eating them raw.

Consume More Glutathione: Glutathione is an antioxidant that will strengthen your immune system and is a pillar in beating Hashimoto's disease. It will boost the body's ability to regulate and modulate your immune system, protects and heals the tissue in the thyroid gland, as well as decrease autoimmune flare-ups. Key foods that will increase the amount of glutathione consumption are asparagus, peaches, broccoli, avocado, garlic, spinach, grapefruit, and raw eggs.

Unknown Food Sensitivities: Those with Hashimoto's disease may have an underlying food allergy that they are unaware of even after consuming the allergen. Upon consuming the food that the individual is allergic too, the antibodies are produced even more so and the thyroid gland is attacked at a higher rate.

Gut Checks: Twenty percent of the functions performed by the thyroid gland depend on the supply of healthy gut bacteria. Taking probiotics will help even out the level of healthy bacteria and will help your body maintain its hormones' balance.

Whole Foods: Eating whole foods will decrease the amount of inflammation. Autoimmunity and systemic inflammation usually work together.

Adrenal Fatigue: There is a connection between your adrenal glands and your thyroid gland. It is uncommon to have adrenal fatigue when you are experiencing hypothyroidism.

Practice Relaxation: Take a look at your life and try to ex out as many stressors as possible. Although it is impossible to rid yourself of all stress, it is important to rid yourself of unnecessary stressors. The thyroid gland is extremely sensitive to the body's stress response. Take up a hobby to relieve yourself of the unnecessary stress and remember to breathe through the small issues that may arise in your daily life.

Thyroid Collar: Unfortunately, life can present situations in which taking an x-ray is unavoidable. Whether it is for the dentist, ER doctor, or another physician, ask for a thyroid collar during your x-ray. The thyroid gland is extremely sensitive to the radiation that is used during x-rays.

Hyperthyroidism

Hyperthyroidism is a condition in which your thyroid gland produced more thyroid hormone (T4) than needed. Common causes of this condition are Graves' disease, abnormal secretion of the thyroid stimulating hormones, inflammation of the gland, excessive iodine intake, or even benign nodules or lumps in the thyroid gland. This condition occurs eight times more so in females than in males. It typically develops in their 30s. However, some symptoms are common in females over the age of 60.

Signs that these may be the issues include weight loss with no explanation, nervousness, irregular heartbeat, changes in the menstrual cycle, excessive perspiration, fatigue, swelling at the base of their neck, difficulty sleeping, and muscle weakness. Although there are other signs, some of the signs are so minor that it is hard to tie them to the condition.

There are ways to treat hyperthyroidism naturally if the condition is relatively new. It is important to see if hyperthyroidism is the cause of some of the conditions that are listed. Untreated hyperthyroidism can lead to other major health conditions. However, if the condition is new then a life style change can help the affected individual and even rid him or herself of this condition.

Bugleweed: Bugleweed is an herb that is also known as *Lycopusvirginica*. It helps control various symptoms experienced from hyperthyroidism. This certain herb reduces the amount of hormones that are produced by the thyroid gland. There have been studies conducted which found out that Bugleweed decreases TSH levels, as well as impairs thyroid hormone synthesis. It helps to lower T4 levels while also blocking the conversion of T4 hormones to T3.

To prepare as a tea; place ½ teaspoon or less of the bugleweed in a cup of water (boiling) and allow it to steep for approximately seven minutes. Strain the bugleweed out of the tea and allow it to cool. Drink this tea once a day.

You are also able to utilize bugleweed as a tincture. You will need to take 2 to 6 ml daily. If you would like to go a step further in the process of ridding yourself of the symptoms relating to hyperthyroidism, then you can make a mixture of bugleweed with a few other ingredients. Use a combination of bugleweed, lemon balm, and motherwort together for an extra powerful, natural tea to help with hyperthyroidism.

Lemon Balm: Lemon balm is also known as *Melissa officinalis.* This is an herb that will normalize an overactive thyroid gland by lowering the TSH levels. Lemon balm contains phenolic acids, flavonoids, and other compounds that are useful to regulate the thyroid gland hormone production.

It works by blocking the active antibodies from stimulating the thyroid gland. This helps those that are suffering from Graves' disease. This herb can be drunk as a tea.

In order to make this tea, add two tablespoon of lemon balm to one cup of water that is boiling. Allow it to steep for six minutes and then strain it. Allow the tea to cool and drink it slowly. You can enjoy this tea three times a day. Should the tea be to strong, you can start off with a lower amount of the herb in your tea and work your way up to the two tablespoons.

Motherwort: Motherwort is an herb also known as *Leonurus cardiac.* This herb acts like a natural beta-blocker. It also helps control your high heart rate and even the heart palpitations. It does include anti-thyroid activity, which allows it to be more beneficial for those who suffer from hyperthyroidism.

In order to prepare this as a tea, steep ½ teaspoon of motherwort in a cup of boiling water for approximately five minutes. Strain the motherwort out of the tea and allow the tea to cool. You are able to enjoy this tea three times a day.

Broccoli: Broccoli does not just serve as a tasty side dish with cheese. It is a cruciferous vegetable that offers substances that are known as isothiocyanates and goitrogens. These help reduce the hormone that is created by the thyroid gland. Those who are suffering from the condition hyperthyroidism will be able to help control it naturally by eating broccoli. The broccoli will need to be consumed raw, as the process of cooking will remove the properties that fight the overactive thyroid. Other vegetables that act the same as broccoli are rutabaga, turnips, cauliflower, Brussels sprouts, kale, kohlrabi, radishes, and mustard greens.

Soy Products: Eating more protein is great for your thyroid functions. Studies performed shows evidence that moderate concentration of sterols in soy will help improve those with hyperthyroidism. If you to not like soy products, you can consume things like nuts, eggs, fish, legumes, and quinoa to produce the same effects.

Omega-3 Fatty Acids: You will experience a hormonal imbalance if you are not consuming enough omega-3 fatty acids. One of the main hormones that this affects include the hormone produced by the thyroid gland called T4. The essential fatty acids are considered to be building blocks for your hormones that ultimately control your immune function, as well as your cell growth. To increase the amount of omega-3, you will need to consume fish, animal products, walnuts, and flaxseeds.

Chapter 6: Natural Ways to Prevent Thyroid Diseases

Diet Changes to Prevent Thyroid Diseases

The thyroid gland is important in our daily and long-term health. Luckily, eating certain products can help keep our hormone levels in balance and our thyroid glands functioning as they should.

Avoid refined food, sugars, saturated fats, and white flour products. Should the thyroid problem be of a severe nature, then it is best to avoid cabbage, broccoli, Brussels sprouts, kale, peaches, pears, and mustard greens. They include anti-thyroid substance and will suppress the functions of the thyroid. (This is typically carried out when hyperthyroidism is the condition at hand.)

Fifty percent of your **diet should be raw and fresh**. Organic and fresh foods are better for your metabolism. The enzymes that thrive in foods help your body in maintaining your metabolism. These foods include salads, sprouts, raw vegetables, and even thermos cooked grains. These foods also help to heal the thyroid gland.

Consume food that are **rich in Vitamin A**. Foods that are rich in vitamin A include eggs, dark green vegetables, and yellow vegetables. It is nature's natural antioxidant producing products.

Each **iodine rich products**. These products include sea vegetables like arame, dulse, kelp, nori, hijike, wakame, or kambu, and fish. These help nourish your thyroid glands and promote a healthy production of hormones.

Copper and zinc are important. These are two key chemicals that is important for a healthy thyroid gland. They help the body produce the thyroid hormone called T4. Foods that can be consumed with these two nutrients in them are beef, oatmeal, seafood, chicken, dried beans, tuna, bran, spinach, nuts, and seed. Foods that specifically include more copper are eggs, yeast, organ meats, nuts, raisins, and legumes.

Consume **more amino acid tyrosine**. Tyrosine is found in chicken, fish, edamame, and beef. Soy should be consumed in small amounts if tyrosine is the nutrients that you are after.

Eat **red and black radishes**. Consuming red and black radishes was actually documented as a real treatment in the Soviet Union for hypothyroidism. The reason for eating radishes is the main sulphur component - raphanin. It is responsible for maintaining the production of calcitonin and thyroxine.

Vitamin/Mineral Consumption for Prevention of Thyroid Conditions

B-Complex: B-Complex aids in improving cellular oxygenation, as well as energy. It builds the adrenals and thyroid. It also calms the nerves of those who consume the proper amount.

Vitamin A: This vitamin assists in keeping the normal functions of your glands balanced.

Vitamin C: This vitamin offers normal adrenal functions, as well as glandular activities.

Essential Fatty Acids: Fatty acids offer glandular health, as well as improve the over all health of those who consume the proper amount. The fatty acids can include omega-3's, as well as 6's. You can consume these by taking in flax oil, flax seed, seed oil, primrose oil, or borage oil.

Multi-Minerals: You are able to take this in a chelated form or liquid form. All the minerals that are involved help glandular health. It helps balance the functions of the glands and in turn helps balance hormone levels.

Calcium/Magnesium: It is important to take in enough calcium and magnesium. These are typically covered in a daily vitamin.

Iodine: You are able to receive the appropriate amounts of iodine by eating iodine-rich foods like kelp or dulse. The correct amount of iodine is 225 to 1000 micrograms daily.

Conclusion

Thank you again for downloading this book!

I hope this book was able to help you to take charge of your own health. Your thyroid gland is important to have a healthy daily life and now you will know what to do and what not to do in order to balance your body.

The next step is to keep yourself motivated on the changes that you will need to complete to be a more energetic person and to have a healthier you.

Finally, if you enjoyed this book, please take the time to share your thoughts and post a review on Amazon. It'd be greatly appreciated!

Thank you and good luck!

www.ingramcontent.com/pod-product-compliance
Lightning Source LLC
Chambersburg PA
CBHW070526290526
45790CB00003B/1318